VET

TOPICS

NAVICULAR
DISEASE

Pablo Adrados de Llano
Álvaro Vázquez-Goyoaga
Raquel Gómez-Lucas

SERVET

Plaza Antonio Beltrán Martínez nº 1, planta 8 - letra I
(Centro empresarial El Trovador)
50002 Zaragoza - Spain

First printing: October 2019

This book was originally published in Spanish under the title:
Síndrome del navicular
© 2018 Grupo Asís Biomedia, SL
ISBN Spanish edition: 978-84-17225-60-5

Translation:
Ubiqus

ISBN: 978-84-17640-96-5
DL: Z 1717-2019

Design, layout and printing:
Servet editorial - Grupo Asís Biomedia, SL
www.grupoasis.com
info@grupoasis.com

GRUPO asis

Servet is the publishing house of Grupo Asís

Warning:

Veterinary science is constantly evolving, as are pharmacology and the other sciences. Inevitably, it is therefore the responsibility of the veterinary surgeon to determine and verify the dosage, the method of administration, the duration of treatment and any possible contraindications to the treatments given to each individual patient, based on his or her professional experience. Neither the publisher nor the author can be held liable for any damage or harm caused to people, animals or properties resulting from the correct or incorrect application of the information contained in this book.

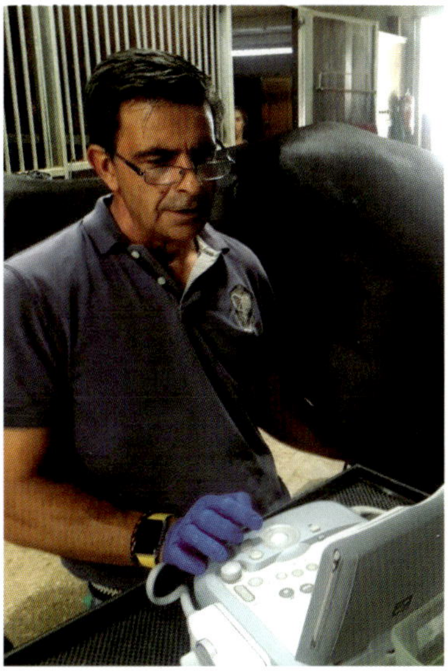

THE AUTHOR

Pablo Adrados de Llano

Degree in veterinary medicine from the Complutense University of Madrid, Spain. The author has been a practicing equine clinician for more than two decades, forming part of the society EQUISAN Veterinaria Equina Integral, of which he is a founding partner. He is a member of the American Association of Equine Practitioners (AAEP) and has served as Chairman of the Spanish Association of Equine Clinical Veterinarians (AEVEE). The author combines his activity in equine clinical practice with teaching. He is the author of the books *Manual para la Determinación de la Edad en el Caballo* (Manual for Determining the Age of Horses) and *Manual de Introducción a la Radiología Equina* (Introductory Manual of Equine Radiology). as well as of numerous informative articles.

COAUTHORS

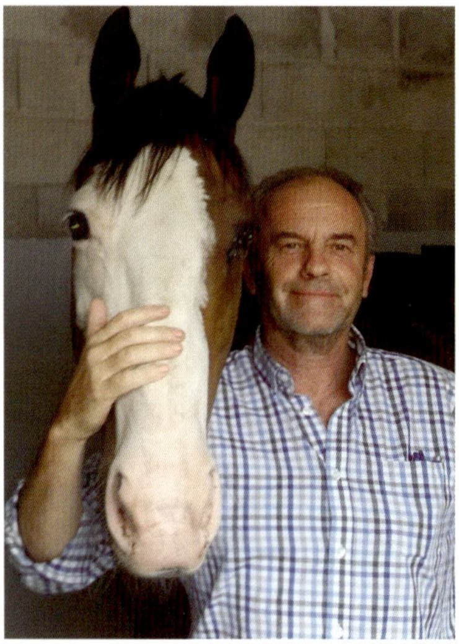

Álvaro Vázquez Goyoaga

Álvaro Vázquez-Goyoaga holds a degree in veterinary medicine from the University of León, Spain (1988). He is specialised and has extensive experience in equine clinical practice, and has worked in all equine sports disciplines. He is particularly dedicated to competition horse medicine and reproduction. He has been a university lecturer since his early days 30 years ago, and is a founding partner of EQUISAN Veterinaria Integral.

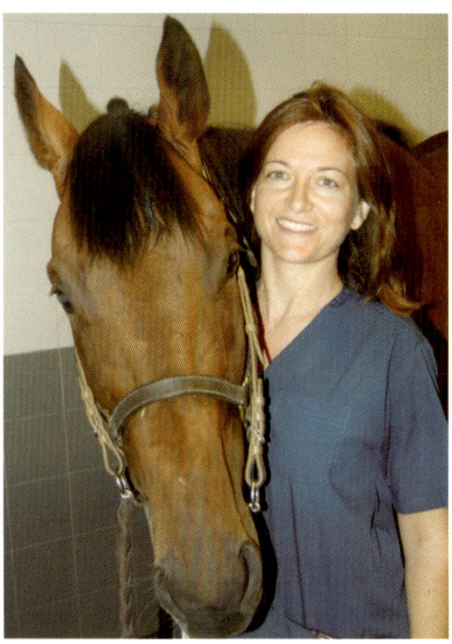

Raquel Gómez Lucas

Raquel Gómez-Lucas holds a degree in veterinary medicine and a PhD in equine sports training and performance. She is certified by the American College of Veterinary Sports Medicine and Rehabilitation (EQ). Raquel Gómez-Lucas has been working at the Veterinary Teaching Hospital of Alfonso X el Sabio University (Madrid) for over a decade, specialised in the field of Sports Medicine and Imaging Diagnosis. She supervises the Department of Magnetic Resonance Imaging for horses of this institution. She combines her clinical work with teaching in various modules of the university's degree in veterinary medicine and master's degree in equine clinical practice. She is author and collaborator of a number of scientific articles and presentations at international congresses.

PREFACE

The podotrochlear apparatus of the horse is the origin of many diseases which in the past, and in the absence of the diagnostic techniques now available, were treated empirically based on the clinical outcomes and experience gained. Nowadays, many of these disorders, which affect a large number of animals, are grouped under the term navicular syndrome, or preferably palmar foot syndrome or podotrochlear syndrome, in reference to a specific type of intermittent chronic lameness involving the structures located in the palmar third of the hoof.

At present, the use of magnetic resonance imaging has allowed us to establish the different bone, tendon, joint or ligament changes that, individually or jointly, lead to lameness and disable or hamper the patient for sports competition.

In this regard, new research lines have been opened, seeking to establish therapeutic and/or prophylactic alternatives that will improve clinical outcomes and avoid the use of multiple treatments which - in the light of our current knowledge of the syndrome - are no longer considered to be justified.

This work provides an update on the existing knowledge of navicular syndrome. It offers abundant information on the clinical findings that can be obtained using different diagnostic tests, as well as on the therapeutic approaches indicated for the different conditions associated with the syndrome, and which in many cases make it possible to successfully prolong the sports life of the affected horses.

Pablo Adrados de Llano

TABLE OF CONTENTS

DEFINITION

Navicular disease is a chronic condition of the forelimbs of the horse caused by alterations of the podotrochlear apparatus (navicular bone and associated ligaments, podotrochlear bursa, deep digital flexor tendon, and distal interphalangeal joint).

This is a chronic and progressive multifactorial disorder which for many years was believed to be of vascular origin, since it caused bone ischaemia and areas of necrosis. The new diagnostic procedures introduced in recent years have shown that injuries in horses with chronic progressive pain in the navicular bone region (Fig. 1) may also implicate other associated structures. Thus, many authors prefer to use the term **palmar foot syndrome** in reference to this kind of lameness.

This syndrome is one of the most common causes of chronic and intermittent forelimb lameness in horses. Since its initial description in 1752 by Jeremiah Bridges, many investigators have attempted to clarify the intricate aetiopathogenic mechanism underlying this disease. While the results obtained to date are not definitive, they offer hope that a full understanding of the disease may be reached over the short to middle term.

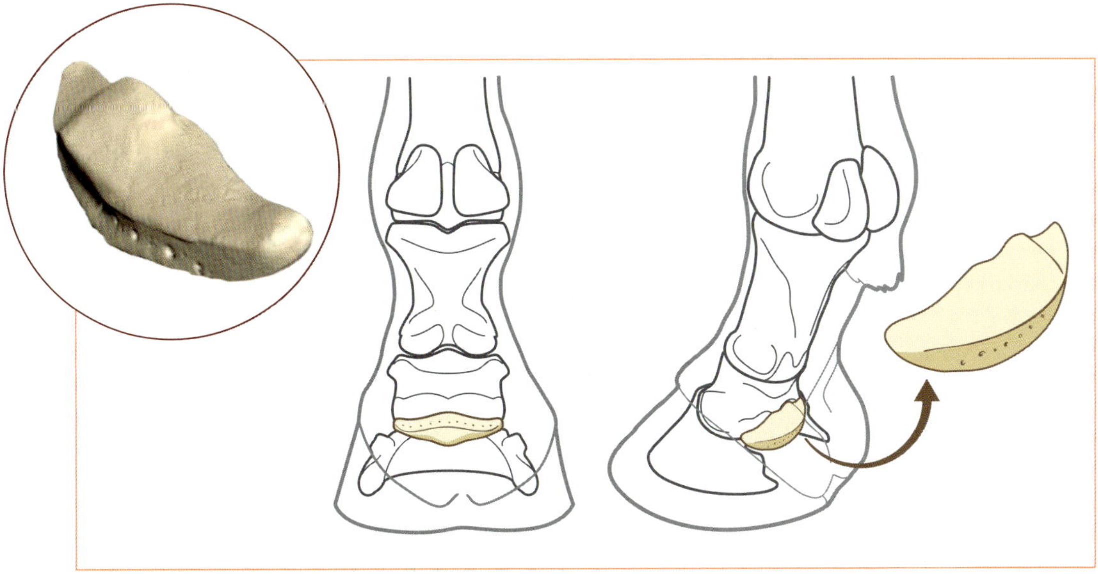

Figure 1. Navicular bone.

ANATOMICAL REVIEW

The navicular bone, also called distal sesamoid bone, is a bone that modifies the direction of the deep digital flexor tendon on its course to insertion into the distal phalanx (Fig. 1). The navicular bone has a proximal margin and a distal margin with nutrient foramina housing small vessels, as well as a medial margin and a lateral margin.

The joint surface presents two depressions for articulation with the distal joint surface of the middle phalanx or crown. The flexor surface, covered by fibrocartilage, is characterised by the presence of a synovial bursa, known as the *navicular bursa*, which connects the margins of the surface with the margins of the opposite surface of the deep digital flexor tendon. The bursa produces synovial fluid, which reduces friction between these two structures. The distal margin shows the development of synovial invaginations that form synovial fossae. The density of the bone is uniform, though the increase in thickness due to the sagittal margin produces a radiological appearance of increased density in this area.

The navicular bone is anchored by three ligaments (Fig. 2):

- Two collateral ligaments (lateral and medial), or navicular suspensor ligaments, that originate from respective depressions located in the distal extremity of the middle phalanx and are inserted on both sides of the proximal margin of the navicular bone following a palmar-distal course.
- A distal (impar) sesamoidean ligament, arising from the distal margin of the navicular bone and running over the flexor surface of the distal phalanx to insert cranial to the deep digital flexor tendon.[1]

There are two synovial structures related to the navicular bone:

- On the one hand, the navicular or podotrochlear bursa, located between the flexor surface of the bone and the deep digital flexor tendon. This bursa extends proximally about 1 cm over the navicular bone and distally to the insertion of the deep digital flexor tendon in the distal phalanx.
- On the other hand, the synovial structure of the distal interphalangeal joint, with a dorsal recess and a palmar recess, extending over the middle phalanx, and a recess between the navicular bone and the distal phalanx.[2]

Although different studies indicate that there is no direct anatomical communication between the aforementioned synovial structures (podotrochlear bursa and distal interphalangeal joint), some authors suggest the possibility of an indirect functional communication. As a result, the outcome of intrasynovial anaesthesia of both the podotrochlear bursa and the distal interphalangeal joint may prove inconclusive.

Arterial blood supply to the bone (Fig. 3) is through the anastomosis between the lateral and medial palmar digital arteries,[3,4,5] which form a proximal plexus with small arteries that penetrate the bone through the nutrient foramina at the proximal margin, and a distal plexus in charge of most of the blood supply to the bone at the distal margin. Some authors have demonstrated anastomoses between both plexuses (proximal and distal).

The main function of the navicular bone is to act as a pulley mechanism for the deep digital flexor tendon. Therefore, the main cause of stress of the bone is the compression exerted upon it by the tendon with each supporting movement of the limb.

In addition, the navicular bone is exposed to compression forces by the second phalanx and suspensor apparatus of the bone itself, i.e. the collateral ligaments and the distal sesamoidean ligament. The degree to which each of these forces affects the bone is determined by multiple factors, though the main contributors are considered to be the weight of the animal and its constitution.[6]

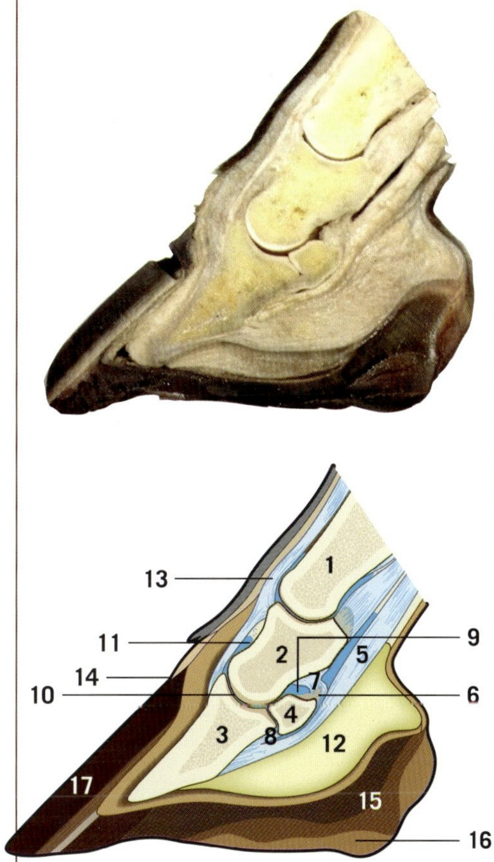

1. First phalanx or long pastern
2. Second phalanx or short pastern
3. Third phalanx or coffin bone
4. Navicular bone
5. Deep digital flexor tendon
6. Podotrochlear bursa
7. Navicular suspending ligaments
8. Distal sesamoidean ligament
9. Proximal palmar recess of the distal interphalangeal joint
10. Distal interphalangeal joint
11. Dorsal recess of the distal interphalangeal joint
12. Plantar cushion
13. Extensor tendon
14. Coronary band
15. Frog
16. Sole
17. Hoof wall

Figure 1. Structures of the podotrochlear apparatus.

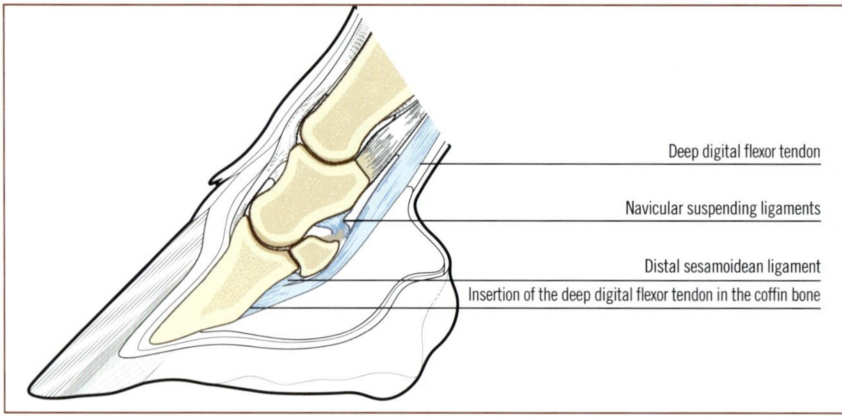

Figure 2. Ligaments and tendons of the podotrochlear apparatus.

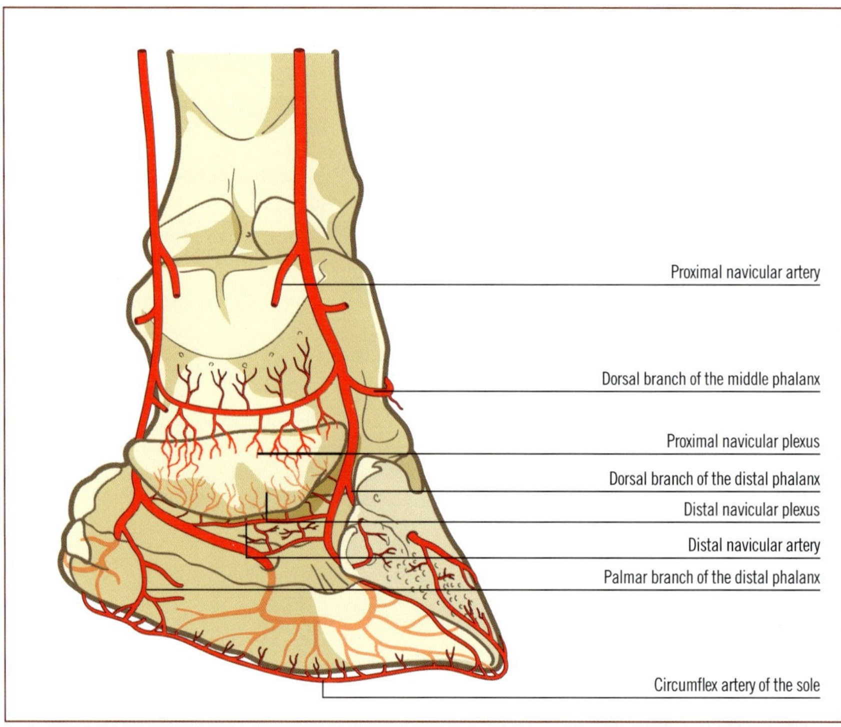

Figure 3. Arterial blood supply of the navicular bone.

AETIOPATHOGENESIS

Because the word "disease" implies a specific cause, the term "navicular syndrome" better describes the aetiology and pathogenic mechanisms giving rise to the clinical signs associated with the navicular bone.

This term should be reserved for bilateral and chronic lameness of the forelimbs, based on a specific diagnostic criterion. However, having clarified this point, we will employ the more widely used term "navicular disease".

Although hereditary causes and breed predisposition have been suggested, the risk factors for the development of navicular bone disorders have not been clearly identified, and the underlying aetiology is speculative.[7] Central European horses are recognised to have a greater tendency to suffer pathological changes (heritability: 0.26–0.3),[8] in the same way as English thoroughbred horses. Likewise, a concave or wavy shape of the navicular bone has been associated with greater alterations than a convex or smooth shape.[9]

In the case of heels that are too low or toes that are too long, or both, excessive pressure may be exerted by the deep digital flexor tendon upon the flexor surface of the navicular bone. According to some authors,[10] such postures alone could cause the disease. It is also common to observe the disorder in the case of hooves that are too small in relation to body weight – this resulting in very high pressures upon the bone within a hoof possessing lesser expansion capacity.

Excessive contusion of the hoof on hard, irregular surfaces also appears to be a predisposing factor. However, it should be noted that the navicular bone is very well protected by ligaments (proximal, distal and lateral), and is supported at palmar level by the deep digital flexor tendon. On the other hand, the disease may also occur in young horses that have been subjected to minimal stress.

Some predisposing factors for the disease include inappropriate postures (Fig. 1) and defective shoeing practices, which can create abnormal forces in the hoof region.

Although adaptive changes in the navicular bone can be found in all horses, pain develops when significant lesions are present.[11]

Repetitive loading cycles may lead to poor functional adaptation and excessive bone remodelling, particularly on the sagittal crest of the bone.[12] Pathological changes often affect the deep digital flexor tendon, in addition to the navicular bone. In fact, changes in vascularisation and in the intratendinous matrix may precede alterations in the flexor fibrocartilage of the bone,[13] and their progression – associated with supraphysiological forces – may lead to erosion of the cortex and trabecular portion, and the development of osteonecrosis and fibroplasia.[14] The final result is the formation of a cystic structure. Concomitant fibrillation of the dorsal surface of the deep digital flexor tendon may occur, forming adherences to the eroded flexor margin.

The vascular theory, postulating hypothetic ischaemic necrosis of the navicular bone, has been ruled out. However, localised pain in this region is related to vascular congestion and increased pressure in the bone and its synovial bursa. In addition, it has been suggested that the increase in distal interphalangeal joint pressure may result in increased pressure within the bursa.[15] It has also been shown that the nerve endings of the collateral ligaments and distal sesamoidean ligament participate in nociception.[5] The arterial blood supply to the navicular bone of a healthy adult horse is characterised by the presence of 48 distal arteries irrigating the central and distal portions of the bone, and 9–14 proximal arteries that cover the proximal portion of the bone. In turn, the lateral and medial portions receive their own arterial blood supply.

Some of the causes of ischaemia of the navicular bone are partial or total occlusion of the digital arteries, arterial obstruction related to arteriosclerosis or thrombosis of the navicular arteries, with resulting venous congestion.

Many theories have attempted to explain the pathogenesis of the disease. In order to facilitate understanding, they will be discussed in relation to the lesions associated with the disorder:

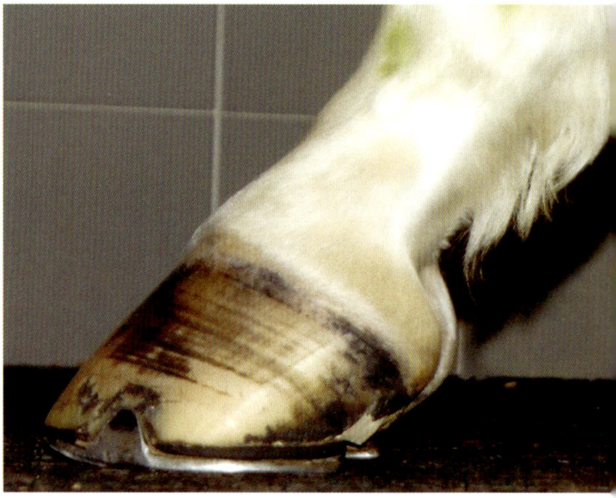

Figure 1. Hoof with long toe and low heel.

PROXIMAL MARGIN

Enthesophytes (Fig. 2) may develop along the insertion of the navicular suspensory ligaments and, less commonly, osteophytes may appear along the proximal border. These lesions are caused by tears in the distal interphalangeal joint or by postural defects leading to excessive pivoting of the navicular bone on its long axis. Following the initial inflammatory response, both enthesophytes and osteophytes are considered to cause no function impairment, though they may favour the development of mild intermittent lameness.

DISTAL MARGIN

The distal margin is characterised by the presence of nutrient foramina and synovial fossae or invaginations. The fossae develop through invagination of the synovial membrane into the nutrient foramen, resulting in widening of the canal containing the artery. The increase in the size of a foramen, with the resulting formation of a fossa, gives rise to the classic radiographic image of the disease, in the form of a lollipop-shaped invagination (Fig. 3). These fossae vary considerably in size, shape, and depth of penetration into the bone. Their primary origin is synovitis of the distal interphalangeal joint. The fossae can be detected in the absence of typical signs of the disease; their diagnostic usefulness is therefore doubtful.

FLEXOR SURFACE

Changes consistent with loss of the fibrocartilage structure are sometimes seen. The presence of diffuse erosions of the surface, leaving the subchondral bone exposed, may be secondary to bursitis/synovitis caused by inflammation of the deep digital flexor tendon in its course over the navicular bone. In addition, adherences commonly develop between the navicular bone and the deep digital flexor tendon, as well as osteitis and ossification of the suspensory ligaments of the navicular bone and of the distal sesamoidean (impar) ligament.

BONE STRUCTURE

It is common to observe areas of diminished opacity in the form of cysts (subchondral cystic lesions [Fig. 4] and sclerosis of the subchondral bone). The underlying aetiology is still unclear, and these lesions are only considered part of navicular disease when related to the sagittal margin of the bone.[16]

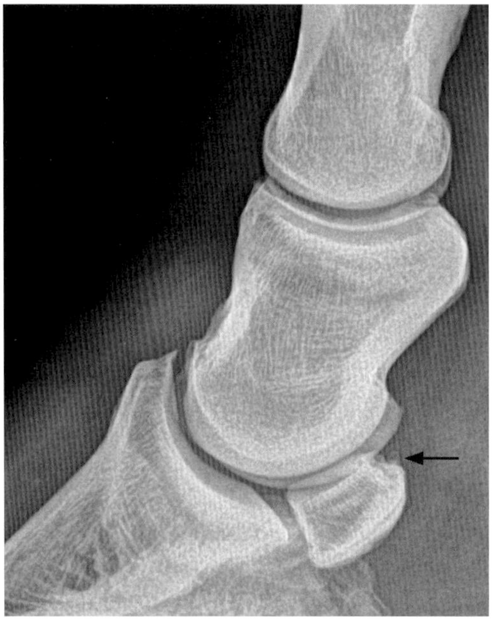

Figure 2. Lateromedial view of the navicular bone: enthesophyte of the proximal margin of the navicular bone.

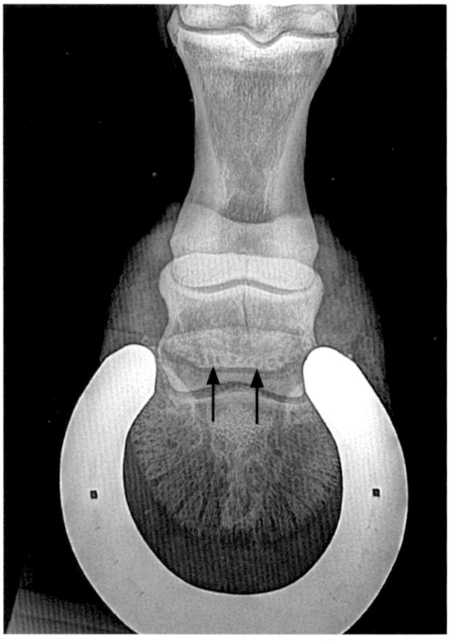

Figure 3. Synovial fossae increased in number and size at the distal margin of the navicular bone.

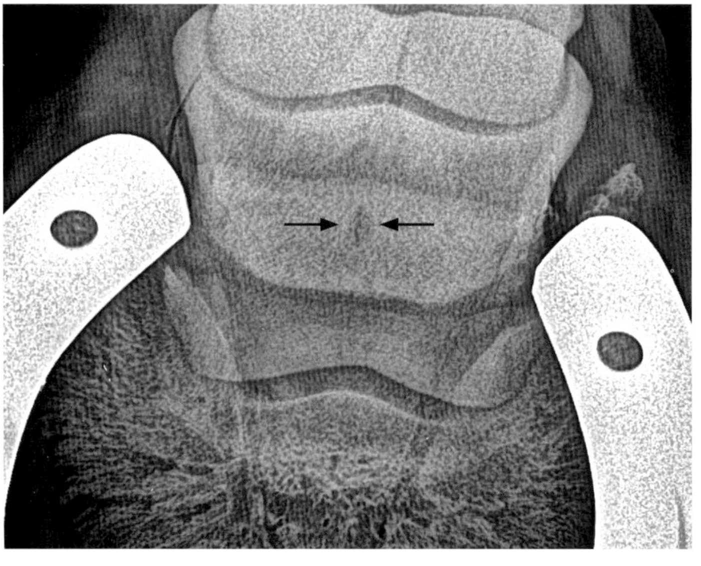

Figure 4. Dorsoproximal-palmarodistal oblique view showing a radiolucent zone consistent with a central cystic lesion of the navicular bone.

Theories for explaining the pathogenesis of navicular disease

1. Vascular origin

The vascular theory suggests that thrombosis of the distal arteries of the navicular bone would cause pain and ischaemic necrosis. This would result in necrosis of the subchondral bone, and reabsorption of the necrotic bone in turn would result in the pseudocystic lesions seen in radiological studies.

2. Biomechanical origin

Changes in conformation and excess loading of the bone (stress) would increase the pressure of the deep digital flexor tendon upon the flexor surface of the bone, leading to degenerative changes in these structures.

3. Degenerative origin

According to this theory, navicular disease would be a degenerative process similar to that seen in osteoarthritis or degenerative joint disease. The changes observed in the bone structure, as well as in the navicular bursa, would be similar to those seen in the hyaline cartilage and synovial membrane of arthritic joints.[17]

It has not been possible to reproduce the disease experimentally. Likewise, the pathogenic relationships between the lesions detected in the bone and the related structures, i.e. deep digital flexor tendon, suspensory and impar ligaments, navicular bursa and distal interphalangeal joint are unclear.

CLINICAL SIGNS

Horses tend to have a history of uni- or bilateral, chronic progressive lameness of the forelimbs. The onset is insidious, and although the disorder is usually bilateral, unilateral presentations can be observed.

While walking or trotting, the horse can be seen to support its weight on the toe region of the hoof in order not to load the zone of the heel. However, in the presence of primary or secondary injury to the deep digital flexor tendon, the horse tends to support its weight on the heels.

The degree of lameness increases when the horse trots in circles, and especially on hard surfaces, being more manifest when the affected limb is the limb facing the inside of the circle. In cases of bilateral involvement, lameness of both limbs is observed on switching hands.

Tests such as forceps pressure (Fig. 1) in the region of the heel, hyperextension of the hoof, or flexion testing are not considered decisive for diagnosing the disorder, since many diseases of these structures can yield positive results with such tests.

In chronic cases, changes in hoof morphology can also be seen, with narrowing of the hoof and increased heel height.

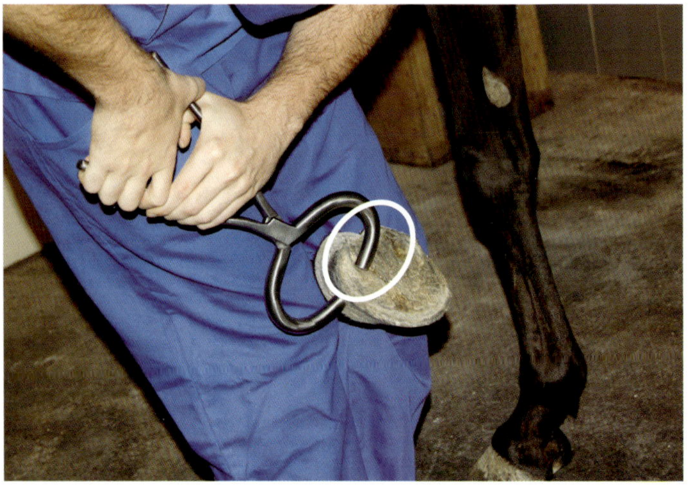

Figure 1. Navicular bone exploration using forceps.

DIAGNOSIS

DIAGNOSTIC ANAESTHESIA

The diagnostic anaesthetic procedures allowing a first approach to the confirmation of navicular disease include palmar digital nerve block and intrasynovial anaesthesia of the distal interphalangeal joint and of the podotrochlear bursa. However, the interpretation of the results of these procedures is complicated, because desensitisation of the structures of the distal third of the limb is unspecific and does not allow for aetiological identification of the pain. Anaesthesia of the palmar digital nerve can desensitise the sole in the dorsal region of the hoof and the distal interphalangeal joint, as well as the heel.[18] Anaesthesia of the distal interphalangeal joint, on the other hand, may cause desensitisation of the bursa and of the navicular bone itself secondary to diffusion of the anaesthetic,[19] relieving the signs in the first 5 minutes. However, a negative response does not exclude podotrochlear disease, because up to 20 % of all cases may prove negative in these diagnostic tests. Similarly, a positive response is not pathognomonic of heel pain. Anaesthesia of the podotrochlear bursa is performed under radiological (Fig. 1) or ultrasound guidance, directing the needle to the middle third of the navicular bone from the proximal side and seeking to avoid inadvertent penetration of the palmar recess of the distal interphalangeal joint or the sheath of the flexor tendons. A positive response after 5 minutes is associated with primary injury of the bursa or the navicular bone,[20] and after 10 minutes it can spread to the distal interphalangeal joint.[19,20] Anaesthesia of the flexor tendon sheath appears to be more specific in detecting lesions of the deep digital flexor tendon or associated structures.

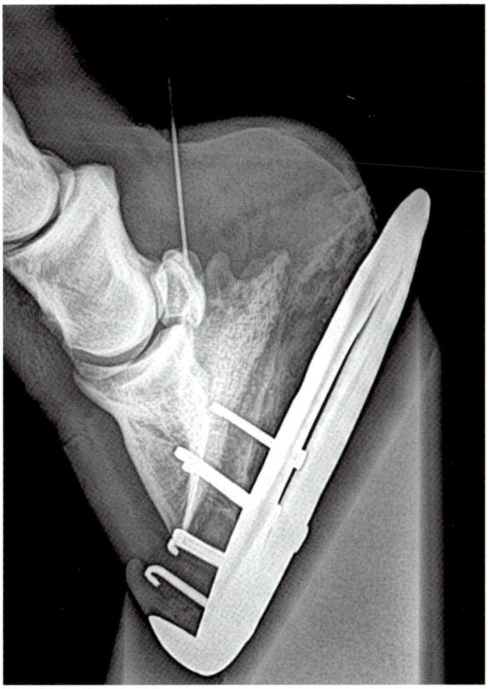

Figure 1. Radioguided injection of the podotrochlear bag.

> Both the volume of local anaesthetic solution administered and the time required to cause the clinical signs to disappear are important factors in diffusion of the anaesthetic and therefore condition the results obtained.

It is therefore advisable to use the smallest possible anaesthetic volume (0.5–1.0 ml axial to each palmar cartilage for blocking the palmar digital nerve; not more than 5 ml for the distal interphalangeal joint; and 2 ml for the podotrochlear bursa).[21] Flexor tendon sheath anaesthesia with 10 ml of 2 % mepivacaine results in some diffusion of the anaesthetic, but the concentrations reached in the adjacent synovial structures are not enough to desensitise the palmar regions, the distal interphalangeal joint or the podotrochlear bursa.[22, 23]

IMAGING DIAGNOSIS

Imaging diagnosis is initially based on radiological evaluation of the hoof. Traditionally, this has been the most widely used method for assessing the internal structures of the horny hoof. However, since more than 40 % of the navicular bone must be mineralised in order for radiographic changes to become manifest, the early degenerative stages may go unnoticed or yield false negative findings.[24] In addition, the results obtained with this technique are variable and often not definitive. In recent years there have been important advances in other complementary imaging modalities such as magnetic resonance imaging (MRI), which have greatly contributed to the diagnosis of multiple disease conditions.

Radiology

Radiographic evaluation of the podotrochlear apparatus requires adequate preparation of the frog zone and correct limb support. It is advisable to remove the horseshoe for optimal visualisation of all the structures. The three most specific radiographic views are:[25]

- Lateromedial view (LM) (Fig. 2): this assesses the thickness of the flexor cortex and its transition to the trabecular portion, the proximal and distal margins of the navicular bone (Fig. 4), and the presence of osteophytes.
- Dorsoproximal-palmarodistal oblique view (DPr-PaDO) (Fig. 3): this identifies the number, shape and position of the radiolucent zones of the distal bone margin, as well as the presence of cystic lesions and enthesophytes at the proximal and distal margins.
- Palmaroproximal-palmarodistal oblique view (PaPr-PaDO 35–50º) (Fig. 4): this detects radiolucent foci adjacent to the palmar surface (Fig. 5), assesses trabecular sclerosis and architecture, delimits the cortical-trabecular transition, and confirms the thickness of the palmar cortex.

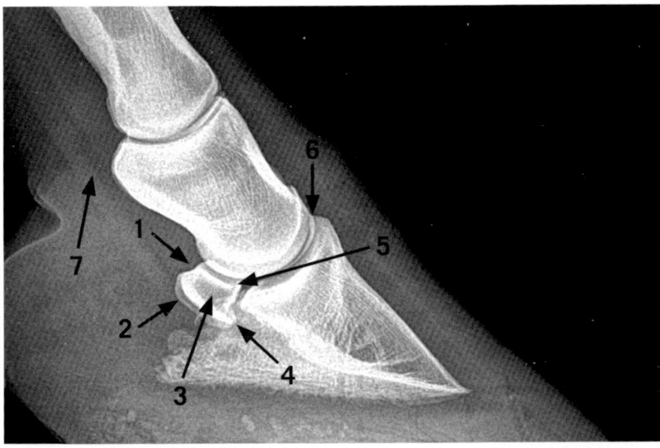

1. Proximal margin
2. Flexor surface
3. Trabecula
4. Distal margin
5. Joint surface
6. Distal interphalangeal joint
7. Deep digital flexor tendon

Figure 2. Lateromedial (LM) view.

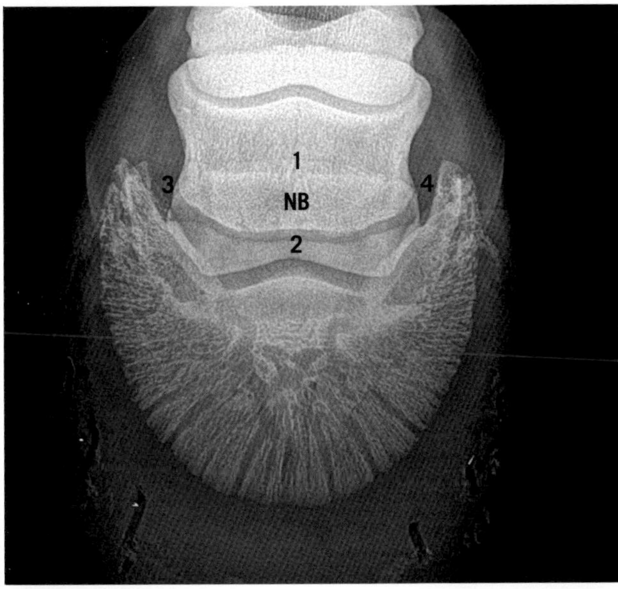

1. Proximal margin
2. Distal margin
3. Lateral margin
4. Medial margin

NB. Navicular bone

Figure 3. Dorsoproximal-palmarodistal oblique (DPr-PaDO) view.

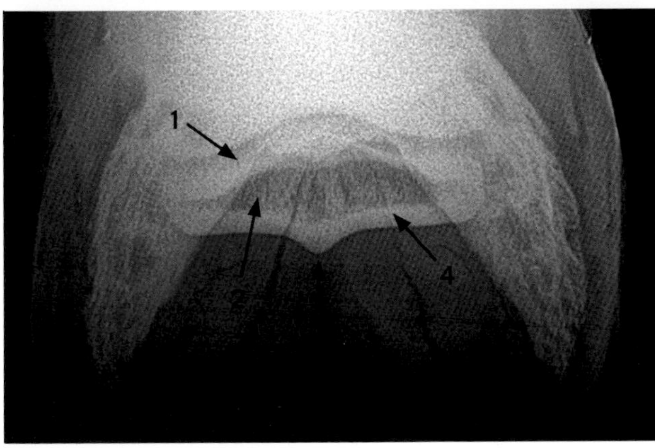

1. Joint surface
2. Trabecula
3. Sagittal margin
4. Flexor cortex

Figure 4. Palmaroproximal-palmarodistal oblique (PaPr-PaDO) view.

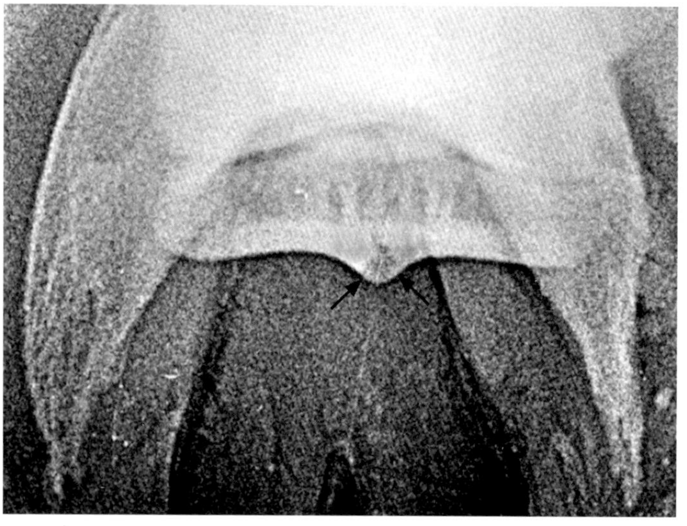

Figure 5. Palmaroproximal-palmarodistal oblique view (PaPr-PaDO): sagittal crest defect of the flexor cortex.

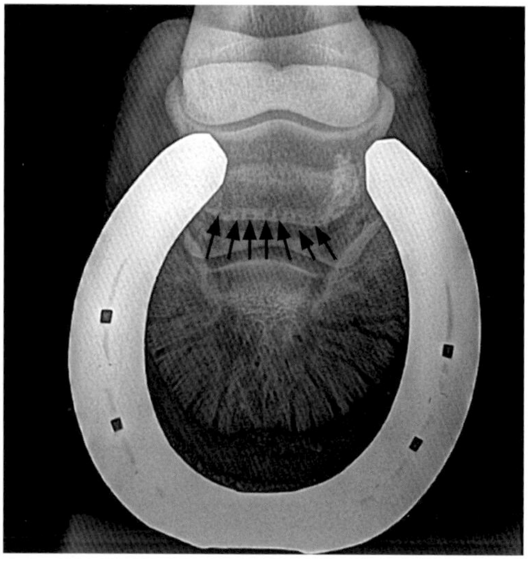

Figure 6. Dorsoproximal-palmarodistal oblique view (DPr-PaDO): multiple radiolucent areas at the distal margin.

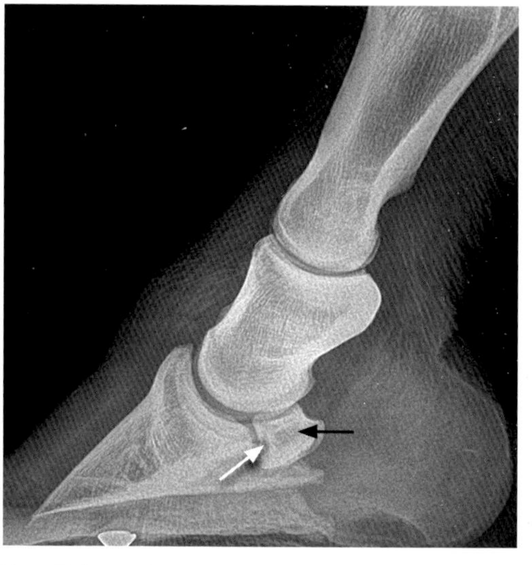

Figure 7. Lateromedial view (LM): loss of cortico-medullary definition (black arrow) and defect at the distal margin (white arrow).

In sum, it is important to assess the presence, number, size, shape and location of radiolucent areas (Fig. 6) at the distal and proximal margins and flexor cortex of the navicular bone, its trabecular pattern, the cortical-trabecular transition (Fig. 7) and the thickness of the flexor cortex, as well as the presence of enthesophytes, mineralisation of the suspensory ligaments, joint osteophytes, and fragments of the distal margin of the bone.

Some concrete circumstances need to be considered, however:

- Although the thickness of the flexor surface of the navicular bone is greater in lame patients than in healthy horses,[24] adult animals usually have a thicker flexor cortex and show a greater presence of enthesophytes at the proximal margin of the bone, not necessarily associated with clinical signs. However, a linear correlation has been demonstrated between the thickness of the compact bone on the navicular flexor side as measured radiographically and injuries of the deep digital flexor tendon, suspensory ligaments, trabecular bone and proximal margin of the bone evidenced by MRI.[26]
- It is accepted that more than 7 radiolucent areas, at both the distal margin of the bone and at its lateral and/or medial margins, predisposes to greater clinical significance. This finding, associated with distal elongation of the palmar surface, may reflect abnormal stress at the origin of the distal sesamoidean (impar) ligament. On the other hand, distal margin fragments at the lateral or medial limits of the bone are an incidental indication of ectopic mineralisation. It is important to take this into account during purchase–sale examinations in order to avoid confusing them with fractures of enthesophyte at the origin of this ligament. However, such fragments are accompanied by clinical signs when they occur associated with a radiolucent area in the distal margin and with numerous synovial invaginations, since dilatation of the latter originates from the recruitment and activation of the osteoclasts around the trabecular nutrient vessels.[6,24]
- Bone resorption at the flexor surface of the third phalanx is described as a focal radiolucent area in the 65° DPr-PaDO view. However, it should be noted that this technique has high specificity (96 %), but low sensitivity (45–55 %) in detecting this finding.[27]
- The radiographic shape of the navicular bone varies among individuals, reflecting the conformation and degree of biomechanical stress to which it is exposed.[28] Horses with podotrochlear disease show very close positioning between the navicular bone and the third phalanx, probably of a congenital nature, which conditions the biomechanical loads supported in this region.[5] On the other hand, hooves with a long toe and a radiographically enlarged angle between the second and third phalanges have a higher incidence of lesions of the trabecular portion and proximal margin of the navicular bone.[26]

Despite the above, no significant relationship between the radiographic findings and the degree of lameness has been established. Among the clinically most representative changes, mention must be made of the presence of pseudocystic formations and trabecular sclerosis, the loss of cortical-trabecular transition, and bone erosion or neoformation at the flexor cortex of the navicular bone.[18] However, the absence of radiographic findings does not rule out the presence of pain associated with the podotrochlear apparatus.

Bursography allows the detection of fibrillation of the dorsal aspect of the deep digital flexor tendon, the formation of adherences between the tendon and the navicular bone, and thinning of the flexor cortex. However, this method has been rendered obsolete by the development of more advanced imaging techniques such as ultrasound and MRI.

Ultrasound

Ultrasound is currently widely used in equine clinical practice, because it offers valuable soft tissue information, particularly in the absence of conclusive radiographic findings. However, it has limitations in application to this anatomical region, due to the horny tissue layer housing all the distal structures. Furthermore, it is difficult to secure an adequate field of view in the presence of contracted or atrophic heels.

The podotrochlear bursa, the proximal margin of the navicular bone, and the distal portion of the deep digital flexor tendon can be accurately assessed[27] adopting a palmar approach through the heel using a 7.5 MHz microconvex probe in longitudinal (Fig. 8) and transverse view (Fig. 9), from the proximal third of the second phalanx to the proximal third of the navicular bone. In distal areas, this procedure can lead to false negative results due to difficulty in securing

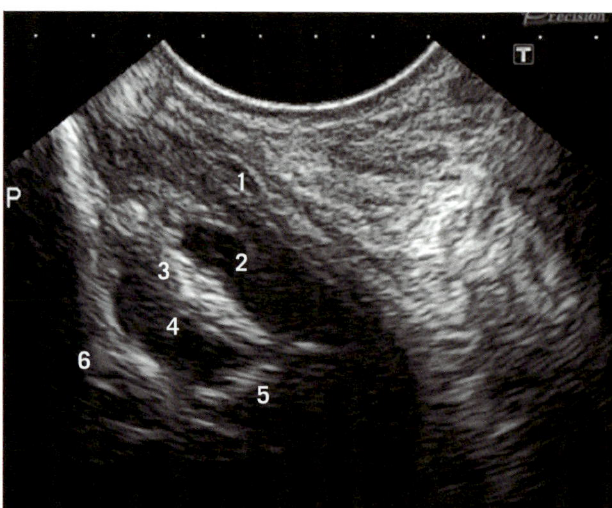

1. Deep digital flexor tendon
2. Navicular bone bursa
3. Proximal collateral ligaments of the navicular bone
4. Proximal palmar recess of the distal interphalangeal joint
5. Navicular bone
6. Palmar surface of the second phalanx

Figure 8. Longitudinal ultrasound of the distal third of the limb. Palmar approach.

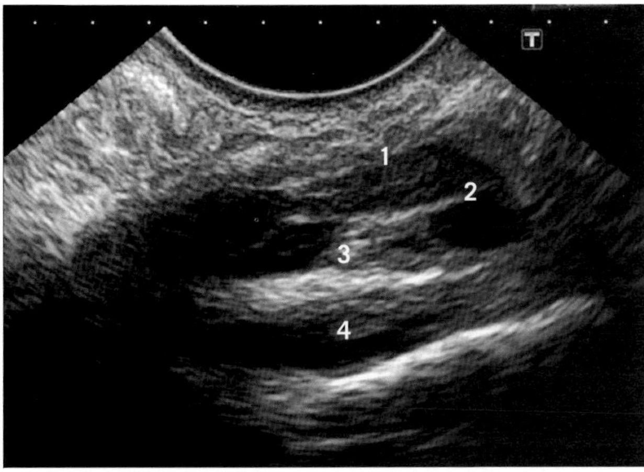

1. Deep digital flexor tendon
2. Podotrochlear bursa
3. Proximal collateral ligaments of the navicular bone
4. Proximal palmar recess of the distal interphalangeal joint

Figure 9. Ultrasound findings related to disease of the podotrochlear system. Palmar approach in cross-sections. Marked distension of the podotrochlear bursa together with the formation of adherences between the dorsal surface of the deep digital flexor tendon, the bursa and the suspensory ligaments.

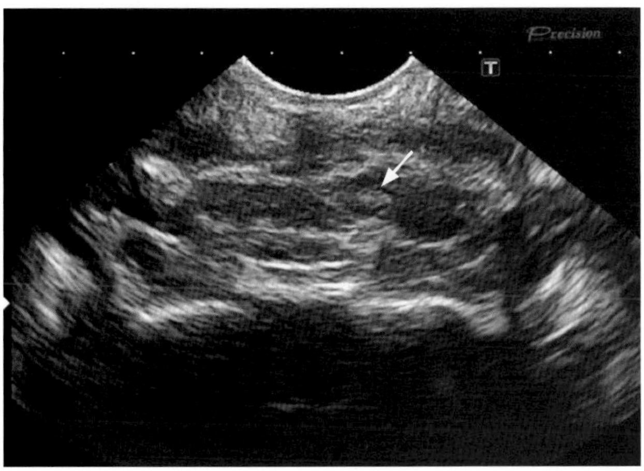

Figure 10. Intratendinous lesion of the lateral lobe of the deep digital flexor tendon.

a correct angle of view of the tendon. As in the case of MRI, we typically observe a series of lesions of the podotrochlear system, with isolated disorders being less common.

Up to 77 % of all tendon disorders (Fig. 10) have been described in the supra-sesamoid region in the lateral lobe of the deep digital flexor tendon in show jumping horses with hoof pain, identified as hypoechoic areas at the dorsal margin of the affected lobe. Ultrasound allows assessment of bursal distension and the presence of internal scar tissue, as well as synovial membrane thickening (Fig. 9). The palmar proximal recess of the distal interphalangeal joint, the suspensory ligaments and the distal digital annular ligament can be assessed in the same way. Distension of the distal interphalangeal joint is also common, and in the same way as with the bursa, it is usually related to other findings in the palmar region.

This technique is more sensitive than radiology in detecting distal interphalangeal joint distension and irregularities of the bony surface of the flexor aspect of the navicular bone (usually associated with deep digital flexor tendon lesions) and of the third phalanx. It is therefore very useful for the early detection of these lesions.[29]

Distension of the flexor tendon sheath is common and nonspecific, and is usually accompanied by injury to the structures it contains. The distal annular ligament can also be related to injuries of the deep digital flexor tendon.[29]

The transcuneal approach through the frog, following due palmar preparation, can detect mineralisation of the distal sesamoidean (impar) ligament, desmopathy of the enthesis of the deep digital flexor tendon over the third phalanx, and changes in the flexor surface of the navicular bone.[30,31,32]

Magnetic resonance imaging (MRI)

This technique (Figs 11 and 12) has become increasingly important in the last two decades thanks to its ability to identify in detail different lesions of the soft tissues, cartilage and bone structures within the hoof. In horses with podotrochlear pain, MRI detects irregularities of the cartilage of the distal interphalangeal joint and subchondral bone, deep digital flexor tendon lesions, desmitis of the suspensory ligaments and distal sesamoidean (impar) ligament, abnormalities of the trabecular portion of the navicular bone and distension of its bursa, among other disorders. This, together with the results of the diagnostic anaesthetic tests, makes it possible to identify many conditions that often appear in combination,[33,34] with a strong correlation to the histopathological findings.[35] Accordingly, today the term navicular syndrome has been relegated in favour of the specific diagnosis of one or more lesions (Fig. 11).

Trabecular lesions of the navicular bone are characterised by a decrease in T1- and T2-weighted signal intensity and an increased intensity in fat suppression (STIR) sequencing. These findings evidence osteonecrosis and fibrosis, oedema with capillary infiltration, degeneration and haemorrhage or fluid-filled cystic spaces at the distal margin of the bone, separated from the synovial invaginations and not necessarily related to alterations of the flexor margin, but which may be concomitant to distal sesamoidean (impar) ligament damage[36] (Fig. 12a).

Erosions of the fibrocartilage of the flexor surface of the navicular bone are more easily detected by MRI than with conventional radiology. The prognosis in relation to return of the horse to competition is usually uncertain; an early diagnosis is therefore required to allow prompt treatment and prevent progression of the disorder. Histologically, these lesions are characterised by degeneration and focal osteonecrosis, and may even affect the trabecular bone. Associated fibrillation of the dorsal margin of the deep digital flexor tendon is commonly observed, [36] giving rise to adherences on the flexor surface and the podotrochlear bursa of the navicular bone in advanced stages of the disease. These findings may be visualised as a simple discontinuity in the synovial compartment, or as the presence of solid tissue between these structures. Synovial inflammation occasionally may be confused with the presence of adherences; the use of contrast medium (gadolinium) is therefore recommended in these cases,[35] or

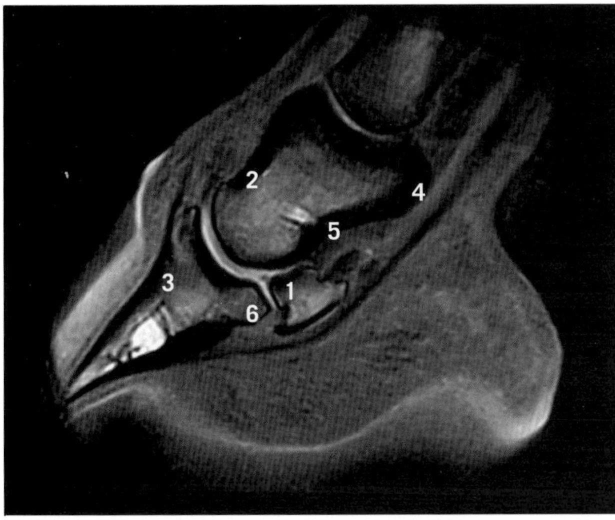

1. Navicular bone
2. Second phalanx
3. Third phalanx
4. Deep digital flexor tendon
5. Proximal collateral ligaments of the navicular bone
6. Distal sesamoidean (impar) ligament

Figure 11. Magnetic resonance imaging view of the distal third of the limb. T1GRE SAG sequence.

bursoscopy to identify the lesions[36] (Figs. 12b and 12c).

Deep digital flexor tendon disease is a lesion commonly detected by MRI (representing 30–64 % of the findings),[37, 38] and its configuration varies over time. Its classification is based on the signal intensity, the affected area and its length and volume, and determines a different course and response to treatment that can be evidenced by performing several MRI studies.[39] Intratendinous lesions may be found in either lobe, as well as longitudinal tears or fibrillation of the dorsal surface with the creation of adherences to the navicular bone and podotrochlear bursa (Fig. 12d).

Resorption of the flexor surface of the third phalanx identified by MRI may appear with age; its clinical significance is therefore doubtful. However, patients with an undesired hoof conformation may develop inflammation in this region, which is rich in sensory nerve endings and arteriovenous complexes, reflecting abnormal stress in the zone. In these cases, it is possible to observe endosteal irregularity of the palmar surface of the third phalanx, cortical disruption, diffuse bone oedema or even the formation of pseudocystic lesions.[36] It is usually related to concomitant lesions of the deep digital flexor tendon and navicular bone (Fig. 12e).

Structural changes in the distal sesamoidean (impar) ligament and suspensory ligaments are usually related to remodelling of the distal and proximal margins of the navicular bone, respectively, as an early sign of bone disease, accompanied by hyperintensity in STIR sequencing,[37] or even a linear signal joining both margins. In more advanced cases, a cystic structure associated with a distal fragment and oedema of the insertion of the distal sesamoidean (impar) ligament can form in the third phalanx.[40] These fragments are not always seen in conventional radiology, MRI and computed tomography (CT) being more sensitive in detecting them. They are clinically more significant when associated with bone changes characterised by large radiolucent areas and enhanced signal intensity in STIR sequencing.[41]

The incidence of primary bursitis and how it is related to the development of pain in the palmar region is not known, since bursal distension

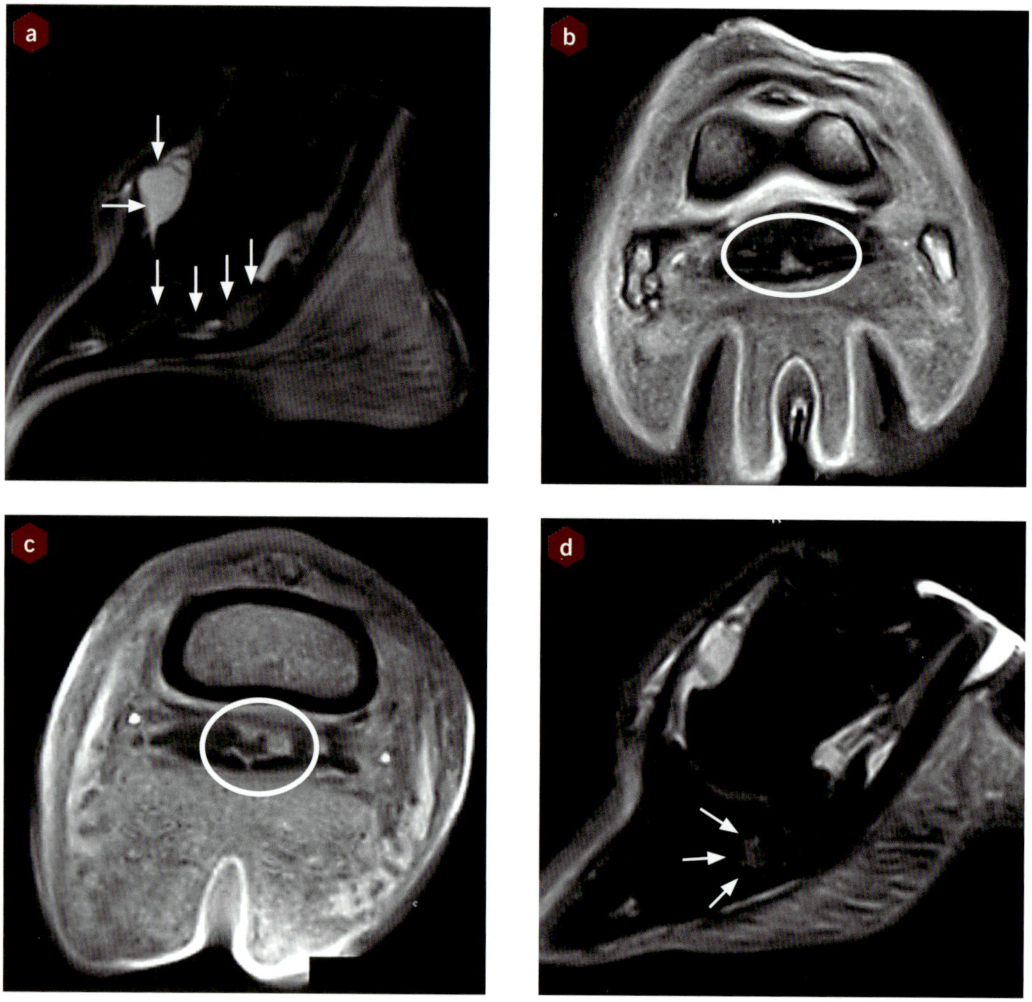

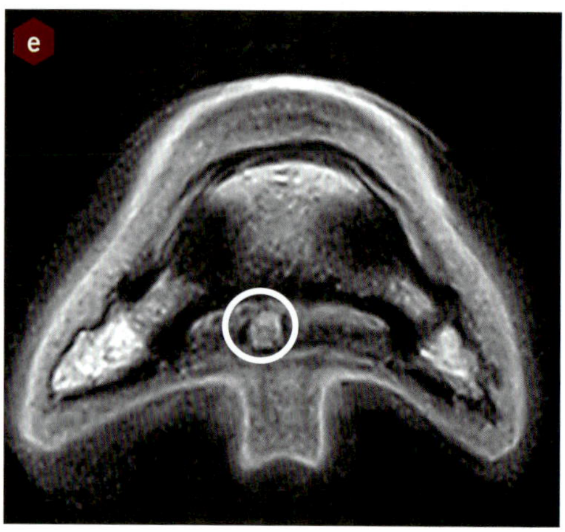

Figure 12. Different findings detected by MRI of the podotrochlear region with the patient in the standing position. (a) STIR SAG sequence. Note the marked hyperintensity of the navicular bone, with more moderate signal intensity of the palmar endosteum of the third phalanx in the region of insertion of the distal sesamoidean (impar) ligament. Note the distension of the proximal recess of the distal interphalangeal joint. (b) T1GRE TRA sequence. Erosion of the fibrocartilage of the flexor cortex of the navicular bone and formation of adherences to the dorsal surface of the deep digital flexor tendon. (c) T1GRE TRA sequence. Region proximal to the navicular bone in the patient of Figure 22b. Note the formation of an adherence to the dorsal surface of the deep digital flexor tendon. (d) STIR SAG sequence. Note the oedema of the palmar endosteum of the third phalanx in the enthesis of the deep digital flexor tendon. (e) T1GRE TRA sequence. Intratendinous lesion in the region of insertion of the deep digital flexor tendon on the palmar surface of the third phalanx.

is a common finding in patients with clinical signs associated with lesions affecting the dorsal surface of the deep digital flexor tendon and the flexor surface of the navicular bone. [41] Hypertrophy and hyperplasia of the synovial membrane, and the associated venous congestion, are related to changes in the suspensory ligaments, distal sesamoidean (impar) ligament or deep digital flexor tendon, with the presence of scar tissue in the most proximal zone of the bursa.[40]

Magnetic resonance imaging frequently allows the identification of combined lesions, though it is unusual to detect isolated individual disorders.[40] It is not clear whether degenerative changes in various structures predispose to concurrent injury, or whether an initial lesion induces instability of all the structures.[41]

Scintigraphy

Increased osteoclastic activity of bone detected by scintigraphy represents a very sensitive but scantly specific finding. This technique may yield false positive findings in healthy horses, as increased radioisotope uptake may reflect biomechanical adaptation in the distal third of the limb. In addition, it may yield false negative findings in patients with signs consistent with podotrochlear pain. However, increased signal uptake in the navicular bone associated with a positive response to intrathecal analgesic testing of the bursa is indicative of a pathological process in this region.[42]

Computed tomography (CT)

Computed tomography is useful for detecting radiographically silent bone disorders in both the trabecular portion and in the flexor cortex, as well as distal fragments of navicular bone.[21] The technique is also useful for characterising lesions of the deep digital flexor tendon with contrast uptake.[43] Its use is conditioned to the availability of such equipment and the need to resort to general anaesthesia to scan the affected region in most hospital facilities (Fig. 13).

Thermography

Thermography is of some use in horses with navicular disease in order to detect potential inflammatory changes in the distal interphalangeal joint. It is regarded as a complementary technique (Fig. 14) in any study of lameness.

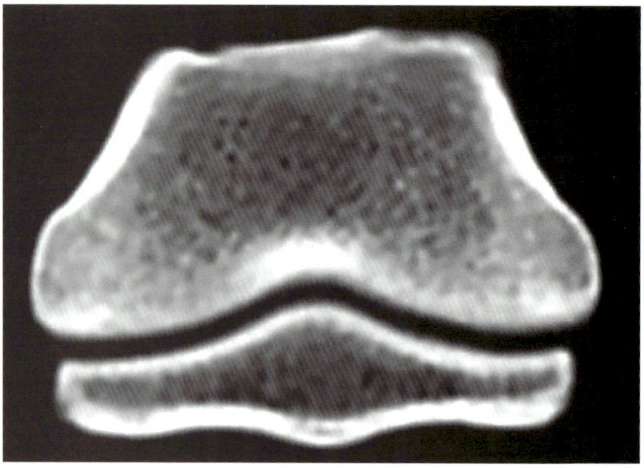

Figure 13. Tomographic image of the normal navicular bone.

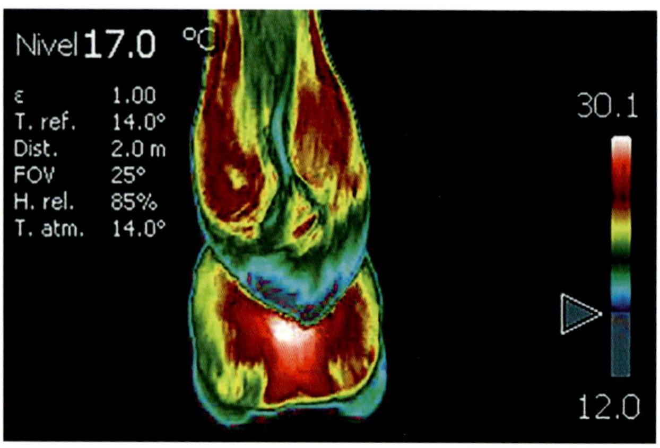

Figure 14. Normal temperature pattern in the navicular zone of a healthy horse.

TREATMENT

In the past, a diagnosis of navicular disease implied withdrawal of the animal from sports life. However, at present, new knowledge about the disease – due in large part to the novel diagnostic techniques used – in many cases allows full recovery of the patient to meet the maximum sports demands.

Nevertheless, there are two types of therapeutic limitations:

- Certain treatments cannot be applied on a regular basis in competing animals due to prohibitions referred to their use. In these cases, strict knowledge of the clearance times is required to ensure maximum performance of horses presenting pain in the podotrochlear area.
- Diagnostic techniques allowing an accurate diagnosis of lesions in the podotrochlear region, with the aim of prescribing the most appropriate treatment, are expensive and not available to all owners. In such cases clinicians, based on their own experience and individual results obtained, tend to establish the most appropriate treatment protocols which, due to the described reasons, are not always the most effective strategies.

The prognosis is largely conditioned by the underlying aetiology. In general, soft tissue injuries and primary lesions of the navicular bone have a guarded and poor prognosis, respectively, in terms of the chances for the patient to return to physical activity.[44]

ORTHOPAEDIC TREATMENT

Trimming and shoeing of the hoof are essential in patients with pain of the podotrochlear apparatus. The main objective of this is to preserve or correct the dorsoplantar and lateromedial balance of the hoof in order to maintain the heel and facilitate lifting of the hoof from the ground.

The shape of the hoof and horseshoe are factors that affect the forces acting in the distal third of the limb.[44] It has been shown that regular intervals in the frequency of shoeing exert palmar shifting of the pressure point and rotation of the distal interphalangeal joint, varying the podophalangeal axis and gradually extending the joint – with an increase in the forces exerted upon the deep digital flexor tendon and navicular bone of up to 20 %.[45] This situation is aggravated when the hoof presents scantly developed heels.[12]

Lifiting of the hoof is facilitated by trimming the length of the toe, moving the breakover point in the palmar direction (by using a rolled toe* [Fig. 1] or setting the shoe back from the toe) or incrementing the dorsal angle of the wall. Likewise, a rolled toe* facilitates lifting of the hoof from the ground, alleviating the pressure exerted by the deep digital flexor tendon on the flexor surface of the navicular bone.[46]

The indications referred to the type of shoe are always related to the identified lesions; a range of possible horseshoes are therefore available on the market.

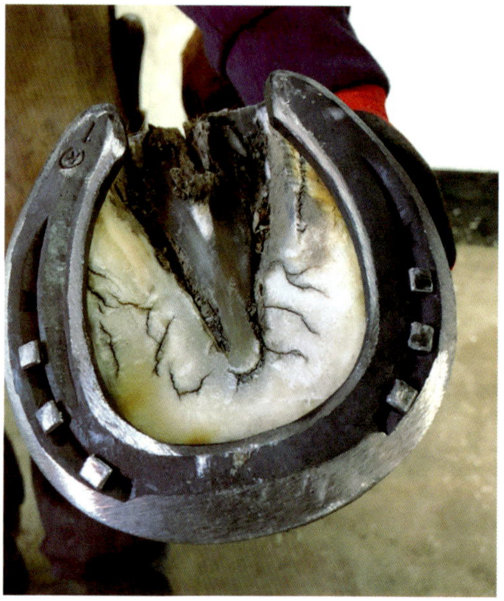

Figure 1. Rolled toe.

Traditionally, it was advised to raise the heels in order to decrease the stress of the deep digital flexor tendon and the forces acting upon the rest of the palmar tissues of the podotrochlear apparatus. However, it should be noted that this therapeutic measure may increase the pressure supported by the articular structures of the distal interphalangeal joint and the podotrochlear bursa.[10] It is therefore recommended that heels be raised by means of a compensated horseshoe or a template fitted to the sole of the hoof in the case of a positive response to hyperextension of the distal interphalangeal joint. Egg bar (or oval) horseshoes increase the contact area and the distance between the shoe toe and the heel, producing caudad displacement of the centre of gravity and reducing the pressure on the navicular bone. This effect is not evident with natural balance shoes or shoes with shoulder tabs.[14]

However, a transition period of 2–3 weeks after shoeing is always recommended to allow biomechanical adaptation, reducing the pain and making it possible to assess the efficacy of the horseshoe.

*Rolled toe: horsehoe that has been rounded on the outer edge of the ground surface at the toe, without modifying the foot surface of the shoe, which is kept flat.

MEDICAL TREATMENT

Nonsteroidal anti-inflammatory drugs (NSAIDs)

These drugs are used as coadjuvants in the treatment of horses with navicular disease. The most commonly used compound is phenylbutazone, which is useful during the acute phase of the disease and provided corrective shoeing has been performed. An adequate treatment regimen consists of 4.4 mg/kg/day of phenylbutazone administered orally until the clinical signs subside, followed by 2.2 mg/kg/day orally until complete remission. Prolonged treatment with phenylbutazone should be avoided due to toxic effects on the gastrointestinal mucosa and kidneys. The effectiveness of flunixin meglumine is similar to that of phenylbutazone, though for cost reasons its use is less widespread. Other NSAIDs used include aspirin and firocoxib.

Intrasynovial medication

Lesions accompanied by distension of the podotrochlear bursa are often treated with intrasynovial injections under radiographic or ultrasound guidance, using a spinal needle from the palmar zone with the limb flexed, which requires crossing the deep digital flexor tendon. Those techniques that approach the bursa from the lateral zone avoid penetration of the tendon.[47,48] However, there is a risk of puncturing the palmar recess of the distal interphalangeal joint or the synovial sheath of the flexor tendons when these are distended. This should be taken into account in cases where bursitis of septic origin is suspected, since there is a risk of accidental contamination of these synovial compartments.

The response to conservative management of the bursa depends on the precise diagnosis of the lesion and how long the pathology has been present. Accordingly, the early detection of lameness (in under 6 months) improves the middle-term prognosis.

The injection of 5–10 mg of triamcinolone provides a favourable response with a view to returning to sports activity, independently of the use of hyaluronic acid. However, the presence of concurrent lesions in the deep digital flexor tendon, navicular bone and podotrochlear bursa implies a guarded long-term prognosis. This is the case of erosive lesions of the navicular fibrocartilage related to adherences of the deep digital flexor tendon and the presence of scar tissue in the proximal recess of the bursa.[38,49]

Both triamcinolone and methylprednisolone (20–60 mg) and betamethasone (3–6 mg) are commonly used, combined or not with hyaluronic acid. They are applied locally in the podotrochlear bursa and concomitantly in the distal interphalangeal joint in those cases where no precise MRI-based diagnosis exists.

Disorders of the deep digital flexor tendon typically have a more uncertain prognosis. Primary tendon lesions respond better to rest and rehabilitation if bursocentesis and an intralesional injection of mesenchymal stem cells and platelet growth factors are performed.[39,50]

Isoxsuprine

Isoxsuprine hydrochloride is a beta-adrenergic agonist with possible vasodilatory and rheological effects that currently is not often used to treat navicular disease. Although its mechanism of action is still unclear, isoxsuprine was found to be effective in the medical treatment of the disease in a clinical trial.[51] Traditionally, two treatment regimens have been used:

- 0.6 mg/kg every 12 hours orally for the first 3 weeks.
- 0.6 mg/kg every 24 hours orally for 2 weeks.
- 0.6 mg/kg on alternate days orally for 1 week more.

- 1.2 mg/kg every 12 hours orally for the first 3 weeks.
- 1.2 mg/kg every 24 hours orally for 2 weeks.
- 1.2 mg/kg on alternate days orally for 1 week more.

Anticoagulant therapy

In the past, anticoagulation was used in an attempt to reduce thrombosis, as ischaemia was thought to be the cause of the disease. Warfarin sodium has been the most widely used anticoagulant. This type of treatment is now seldom used due to its weak scientific basis and because of the severe side effects that may occur.

Bisphosphonates

Changes related to bone remodelling in navicular disease have been widely described and include bone resorption evidenced as transparent areas on radiographs, subchondral sclerosis, and bone neoformation in the ligament attachment zones at the proximal margin of the navicular bone.[52] Bisphosphonates, as shown in different experimental studies in humans and animals, bind to calcium and other divalent ions in the bloodstream and are deposited in the active remodelling zones of different sites, inhibiting osteoclast recruitment, adhesion, differentiation and resorptive activity. Although their half-life in blood is short, bisphosphonates rapidly accumulate in bone, where they remain for long periods of time subject to bone turnover – with the active drug being released into the bone remodelling zone.[52]

Parenteral bisphosphonates (disodium clodronate or tiludronate) are indicated when bone resorption or remodelling of navicular bone is detected.[53,54]

Although these drugs have been considered to produce an initial analgesic effect, the response to treatment is highly variable and dependent upon the diagnosis of the lesion associated with the bone structure. Navicular bone resorption is only seen radiographically once over 40 % of normal bone structure has been lost. The use of other more advanced and sensitive imaging techniques, such as MRI or CT, therefore facilitates the identification of possible changes in the navicular bone and the indication of bisphosphonate use.

The administration of disodium tiludronate has been shown to be effective at doses of 0.1 mg/kg administered intravenously for 10 days. However, it appears that better responses are obtained with a single intravenous dose of 1 mg/kg, diluted in saline solution over a period of 30 minutes. Tiludronate has also been administered as a regional intravenous infusion involving a single 0.1 mg/kg dose into the palmar digital vein, with the obtainment of different results.

Recently introduced for use in horses with navicular disease, disodium clodronate has been used in a study[55] as a single intramuscular dose of 1.4 mg/kg (60 mg/ml) at three different points, equivalent to 1.19 mg/kg of clodronic acid – a positive response being recorded in 67 % of the treated horses versus in 21 % of the horses in the placebo group (Table 1).

Table 1. Positive response (95 % confidence interval [95 %CI]) during the study.[55]

	Number of horses (n)		Positive response (%) (95 %CI)	
	Clodronate	**Placebo**	**Clodronate**	**Placebo**
Day 28	89	29	67 % (58–77 %)	21 % (6–35 %)
Day 56	86	28	75 %[a] (35–94%)	3 % (0.3–26 %)
Day 180	61	NA[b]	84 % (74–93 %)	NA[b]

[a] Significantly different (p=0.003) from placebo. [b] Nonapplicable/nonevaluable controls due to compassionate use of treatment after day 56.

Bursoscopy

Lameness associated with bursitis of the navicular bone is usually accompanied by tendon lesions. The inclusion criteria considered for performing podotrochlear bursa endoscopy are the presence of lameness located in the hoof, the absence of significant radiographic lesions in the navicular bone, and a positive response to anaesthesia of the podotrochlear bursa, or the existence of MRI images consistent with intrathecal bursa injury.[56] In some cases, the only criterion for performing bursoscopy is a positive response to anaesthesia of the podotrochlear bursa, even if no abnormalities are detected by MRI.

Bursoscopy is an invasive technique that facilitates specific visualisation and treatment of adherences among the fibrocartilage of the flexor surface of the navicular bone, the podotrochlear bursa, and the dorsal aspect of the deep digital flexor tendon.[57] The prognosis after debridement depends on the severity of the initial injury, but is usually better than with conservative treatment[56] (Fig. 2).

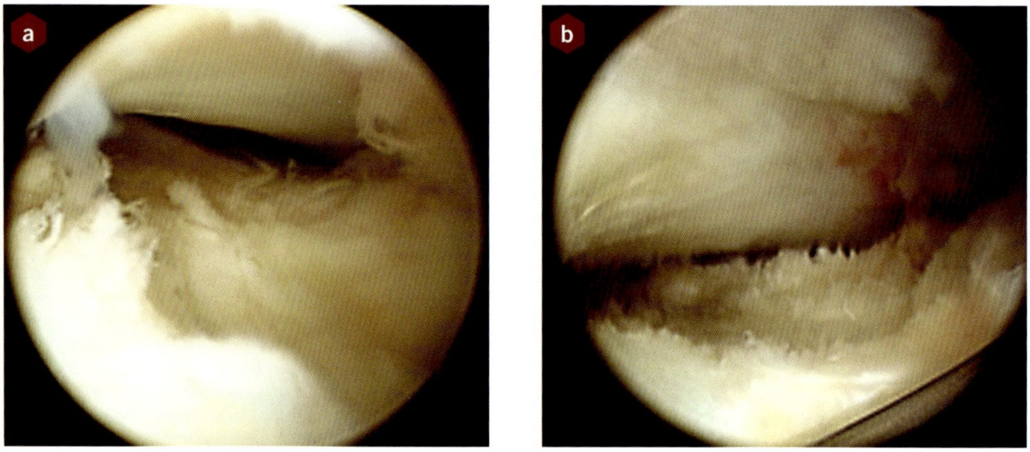

Figure 2. Endoscopic appearance of the inside of the podotrochlear bursa showing (a) fibrillation of the dorsal surface of the deep digital flexor tendon; and (b) erosion of the fibrocartilage of the flexor cortex.

Extracorporeal shock wave therapy (ESWT)

This is a noninvasive treatment modality involving the application of high-frequency sound waves to the tissues. Although the mechanism of action of ESWT has not been clearly established, the technique appears to promote neovascularisation of the tendon-to-bone enthesis and provides an analgesic effect by decreasing neuronal transmission of local nociceptive stimuli when applied through the heel.[58]

SURGICAL TREATMENT

Surgery should be reserved for cases failing to respond to medical treatment.

Palmar digital neurectomy

Neurectomy of the lateral and medial palmar digital nerves, as well as of their collateral branches, is the most effective technique in patients with navicular disease failing to respond to medical treatment. It is only useful when anaesthetic block of these nerves at the mid-pastern level is clearly positive. This technique results in desensitisation of the caudad third of the hoof, including the navicular bone. The operation can be performed with the animal in standing position using only local anaesthesia, or under general anaesthesia (the latter option is advised). Transection of the nerve can be performed with or without epineural capping*; the former approach reduces the possibility of nerve regeneration and therefore of subsequent neuroma formation.

*Epineural capping: a surgical procedure in which the proximal end of a sectioned nerve is enveloped in epineurium to prevent the formation of neuromas.

Neurectomy is contraindicated in cases of deep digital flexor tendon injuries, because the tendon might rupture with normal movement of the hoof.

The complications that may occur after neurectomy mainly include neuromas, rupture of the deep digital flexor tendon, and loss of blood supply to the hoof secondary to fibrosis of the zone. In the latter two cases euthanasia is recommended, while neuroma formation requires a new neurectomy above the affected site.

Despite the complications associated to the technique, some horses may not present lameness for up to 5 years after neurectomy.[59]

Desmotomy of the suspensory ligaments of the navicular bone

This technique is now seldom used, due to the scant results obtained in horses with flexor cortex defects, mineralisation of the deep digital flexor tendon, and medullary sclerosis.[58] Desmotomy is sometimes used adopting an arthroscopic approach to the palmar aspect of the distal interphalangeal joint in horses with primary lesions of the collateral ligament of the navicular bone.[51]

REFERENCES

1. Baxter GM. *Adams and Stashak's Lameness in Horses.* 6th edition. Miley-Blackwell. 2011; 242–245.
2. Kainer RA. Clinical anatomy of the equine foot. *Vet Clin North Am Equine Pract.* 1989; 5:1–27.
3. Pool RR, Meagher DM, Stover SM. Pathophysiology of navicular syndrome. *Vet Clin North Am Equine Pract.* 1989; 5:109–129.
4. Pleasant RS, Chrisman MC. Navicular disease in horses: pathogenesis and diagnosis. *Vet Med.* 1997; 250-257.
5. Bowker RM, Linder K, VanWalfen KK et al. Distribution of local anesthetic injected into the distal interphalangeal joint and podotrochlear bursa: an experimental study. *Pferdeheilkunde.* 1996; 609–612.
6. Wright IM, Douglas J. Biomechanical considerations in the treatment of navicular disease. *Vet Rec.* 1993; 133:109–114.
7. Stock KF, Hamann H, Distl O. Variance component estimation on the frequency of pathologic changes in the navicular bones of Hanoverian Warmblood horses. *J Anim Breed Genet.* 2004; 121(5):289–301.
8. van den Belt AJ, Dik KJ and van den Broek J. The use of radiography as a tool for the efficacy of selective breeding of a poor radiographic navicular bone condition (grades 3 and 4). *Proc 13th Int Vet Radio*, South Africa. 2003.
9. Dik KJ, van den Belt AJ, van den Broek J. Relationships of age and shape of the navicular bone to the development of navicular disease: a radiological study. *Equine Vet J.* 2001; 33(2):172–175.
10. Rooney JR. The foreleg. In: *The Mechanics of the Horse.* Malabar, FL, Robert E. Kreiger. 1980; 60–61.
11. Blunden A, Dyson S, Murray R et al. Histopathology in horses with chronic palmar foot pain and age-matched controls. Part 1: Navicular bone and related structures. *Equine Vet J.* 2006; 38(1):15–22.
12. Bentley VA, Sample SJ, Livesey MA et al. Morphologic changes associated with functional adaptation of the navicular bone of horses. *J Anat.* 2007; 211(5):662–672.
13. Blunden A, Dyson S, Murray R et al. Histopathology in horses with chronic palmar foot pain and age-matched controls . Part 2: The deep digital flexor tendon. *Equine Vet J.* 2006; 38:23–27.
14. Sherlock C, Mair T, Blunden T. Deep erosions of the palmar aspect of the navicular bone diagnosed by standing magnetic resonance imaging. *Equine Vet J.* 2008; 40(7):684–692.
15. Viitanen MJ, Wilson AM, McGuigan HR et al. Effect of foot balance on the intra-articular pressure in the distal interphalangeal joint in vitro. *Equine Vet J.* 2003; 35:184–189.
16. Butler J, Colles C, Dyson S et al. In: *Foot, pastern and fetlock. Clinical Radiology of the Horse.* 2nd edition. Oxford, Blackwell Scientific. 2000; pp. 27–130.

17. Pool RR, Meagher DM, Stover SM. Pathophysiology of navicular syndrome. *Vet Clin North Am Equine Pract.* 1989; 5:109–129.
18. Ross MW and Dyson SJ. *Diagnosis and Management of Lameness in the Horse.* 2nd edition. Saunders. 2011.
19. Schumacher J, Schumacher J, Gillette R et al. The effects of local anaesthetic solution in the navicular bursa of horses with lameness caused by distal interphalangeal joint pain. *Equine Vet J.* 2003; 35(5):502–505.
20. Crowe OM, Hepburn RJ, Kold SE et al. Long-term outcome after arthroscopic debridement of distal phalanx extensor process fragmentation in 13 horses. *Vet Surg.* 2010; 39(1):107–114.
21. Rijkenhuizen AB. Navicular disease: a review of what's new. *Equine Vet J.* 2006; 38:82–88.
22. Harper J, Schumacher J, DeGraves F et al. Effects of analgesia of the digital flexor tendon sheath on pain originating in the sole, distal interphalangeal joint or navicular bursa of horses. *Equine Vet J.* 2007; 39(6):535–539.
23. Jordana M, Martens A, Duchateau L et al. Diffusion of mepivacaine to adjacent synovial structures after intrasynovial analgesia of the digital flexor tendon sheath. *Equine Vet J.* 2015; 48:326–330.
24. Biggi M, Dyson S. Distal border fragments and shape of the navicular bone: Radiological evaluation in lame horses and horses free from lameness. *Equine Vet J.* 2012; 44(3):325–331.
25. Dyson S. Radiological interpretation of the navicular bone. *Equine Vet Educ.* 2011; 23(2):73–87.
26. de Zani D, Polidori C, di Giancamillo M et al. Correlation of radiographic measurements of structures of the equine foot with lesions detected on magnetic resonance imaging. *Equine Vet J.* 2015; 165–171.
27. Young AC, Dimock AN, Puchalski SM et al. Magnetic resonance and radiographic diagnosis of osseous resorption of the flexor surface of the distal phalanx in the horse. *Equine Vet J.* 2012; 44(suppl. 43):3–7.
28. Kaser-Hotz B, Ueltschi G. *Radiographic appearance of the navicular bone in sound horses. Vet Radiology and Ultrasound.* Blackwell Publishing Ltd. 1992; 33(1):9–17.
29. Rabba S, Bolen G, Verwilghen D et al. Ultrasonographic Findings In Horses With Foot Pain But Without Radiographically Detectable Osseous Abnormalities. *Vet Radiol Ultrasound.* 2011; 52(1):95–102.
30. Busoni V, Denoix J. Ultrasonography of the Podotrochlear Apparatus in the Horse Using a Transcuneal Approach: Technique and Reference Images. *Vet Radiol Ultrasound.* 2001; 42(6):534–540.
31. Grewal JS, McClure SR, Booth LC et al. Assessment of the ultrasonographic characteristics of the podotrochlear apparatus in clinically normal horses and horses with navicular syndrome. *J Am Vet Med Assoc.* 2004; 225(12):1881–1888.

32. Bolen G, Busoni V, Jacqmot O et al. Sonographic anatomy of the palmarodistal aspect of the equine digit. *Vet Radiol Ultrasound.* 2007; 48(3):270–275.
33. Sampson SN, Schneider RK, Gavin PR et al. Magnetic resonance imaging findings in horses with recent onset navicular syndrome but without radiographic abnormalities. *Vet Radiol Ultrasound.* 2009; 50(4):339–346.
34. Murray RC, Schramme MC, Dyson SJ et al. Magnetic resonance imaging characteristics of the foot in horses with palmar foot pain and control horses. *Vet Radiol Ultrasound.* 2006; 47(1):1–16.
35. Murray RC, Blunden TS, Schramme MC et al. How does magnetic resonance imaging represent histologic findings in the equine digit? *Vet Radiol Ultrasound.* 2006; 47(1):17–31.
36. Busoni V, Heimann M, Trenteseaux J et al. Magnetic resonance imaging findings in the equine deep digital flexor tendon and distal sesamoid bone in advanced navicular disease – An ex vivo study. *Vet Radiol Ultrasound.* 2005; 46(4):279–286.
37. Dyson SJ, Murray R, Schramme MC. Lameness associated with foot pain: results of magnetic resonance imaging in 199 horses (January 2001–December 2003) and response to treatment. *Equine Vet J.* 2005; 37(2):113–121.
38. Bell CD, Howard RD, Taylor DS et al. Outcomes of podotrochlear (navicular) bursa injections for signs of foot pain in horses evaluated via magnetic resonance imaging: 23 cases (2005–2007). *J Am Vet Med Assoc.* 2009; 234(7):920–925.
39. Vanel M, Olive J, Gold S et al. Clinical significance and prognosis of deep digital flexor tendinopathy assessed over time using MRI. *Vet Radiol Ultrasound.* 2012; 53(6):621–627.
40. Dyson S, Pool R, Blunden T et al. The distal sesamoidean impar ligament: Comparison between its appearance on magnetic resonance imaging and histology of the axial third of the ligament. *Equine Vet J.* 2010; 42(4):332–9.
41. Biggi M, Dyson S. High-field magnetic resonance imaging investigation of distal border fragments of the navicular bone in horses with foot pain. *Equine Vet J.* 2011; 43(3):302–308.
42. Dyson SJ. Subjective and quantitative scintigraphic assessment of the equine foot and its relationship with foot pain. *Equine Vet J.* 2002; 34:164–170.
43. Nelson BB, Goodrich LR, Barrett MF et al. Use of contrast media in computed tomography and magnetic resonance imaging in horses: Techniques, adverse events and opportunities. *Equine Vet J.* 2017; 49(4):410–424.
44. Parkes RSV, Witte TH. The foot-surface interaction and its impact on musculoskeletal adaptation and injury risk in the horse. *Equine Vet J.* 2015; 47:519–525.
45. Moleman M, van Heel MC, van Weeren PR et al. Hoof growth between two shoeing sessions leads to a substantial increase of the moment about the distal, but not the proximal, interphalangeal joint. *Equine Vet J.* 2006; 38(2):170–174.

46. van Heel MC, van Weeren PR, Back W. Shoeing sound warmblood horses with a rolled toe optimises hoof-unrollment and lowers peak loading during breakover. *Equine Vet J.* 2006; 38:258–262.
47. Daniel AJ, Goodrich LR, Barrett MF et al. An optimised injection technique for the navicular bursa that avoids the deep digital flexor tendon. *Equine Vet J.* 2015; (1):159–164.
48. Nottrott K, De Guio C, Khairoun A et al. An ultrasound-guided, tendon-sparing, lateral approach to injection of the navicular bursa. *Equine Vet J.* 2017; 49(5):655–661.
49. Marsh CA, Schneider RK, Sampson SN et al. Response to injection of the navicular bursa with corticosteroid and hyaluronan following high-field magnetic resonance imaging in horses with signs of navicular syndrome: 101 cases (2000–2008). *J Am Vet Med Assoc.* 2012; 241(10):1353–1364.
50. Gutierrez-Nibeyro SD, White NA, Werpy NM. Outcome of medical treatment for horses with foot pain: 56 cases. *Equine Vet J.* 2010; 42(8):680–685.
51. Turner AS, Tucker CM. The evaluation of isoxsuprine hydrochloride for the treatment of navicular disease: a double blind study. *Equine Vet J.* 1989; 21:338–341.
52. McLellan J. Science-in-brief: Bisphosphonate use in the racehorse: Safe or unsafe? *Equine Vet J.* 2017; 49(4):404–407.
53. Denoix JM, Thibaud D, Riccio B. Tiludronate as a new therapeutic agent in the treatment of navicular disease: a double-blind placebo-controlled clinical trial. *Equine Vet J.* 2003; 35(4):407–413.
54. Whitfield CT, Schoonover MJ, Holbrook TC et al. Quantitative assessment of two methods of tiludronate administration for the treatment of lameness caused by navicular syndrome in horses. *Am J Vet Res.* 2016; 77(2):167–173.
55. Frevel M, King BL, Kolb DS et al. Clodronato disódico para el tratamiento de los signos clínicos de enfermedad navicular – un ensayo clínico doble ciego, controlado con placebo. *Pferdeheilkunde.* 2017; 33(2):271–279.
56. Smith MRW, Wright IM. Endoscopic evaluation of the navicular bursa: Observations, treatment and outcome in 92 cases with identified pathology. *Equine Vet J.* 2012; 44(3):339–345.
57. Smith MRW, Wright IM, Smith RKW. Endoscopic assessment and treatment of lesions of the deep digital flexor tendon in the navicular bursae of 20 lame horses. *Equine Vet J.* 2007; 39(1):18–24.
58. Bolt DM, Burba DJ, Hubert JD et al. Determination of functional and morphologic changes in palmar digital nerves after nonfocused extracorporeal shock wave treatment in horses. *Am J Vet Res.* 2004; 65(12):1714–1718.
59. Gutierrez-Nibeyro SD, Werpy NM, White NA et al. Outcome of palmar/plantar digital neurectomy in horses with foot pain evaluated with magnetic resonance imaging: 50 cases (2005–2011). *Equine Vet J.* 2015; 47(2):160–164.